SIMPLY KETO COMFORT FOODS WORKBOOK

by

Marie Emmerich

LIVE

LOVE

KETO

Track Your Progress

Day .... Date.................

- ## Diet Plan

  ....
  ....
  ....

- ## How do you feel?

  ....
  ....
  ....
  ....

- ## Record your weight: ....

Track Your Progress

Day .... Date.................

- ### Diet Plan

  ....
  ....

- ### How do you feel?

  ....
  ....
  ....

- **Record your weight:** ....

Track Your Progress

Day ....   Date.................

- ## Diet Plan

....
....
....

- ## How do you feel?

....
....
....
....

- **Record your weight:** ....

Track Your Progress

Day .... Date..................

- ## Diet Plan

....
....

- ## How do you feel?

....
....
....

- ## Record your weight: ....

Track Your Progress

Day ....   Date.................

- ## Diet Plan

  ....
  ....
  ....

- ## How do you feel?

  ....
  ....
  ....
  ....

- ## Record your weight: ....

<u>Track Your Progress</u>

Day .... **Date**.................

- ## <u>Diet Plan</u>

  ....
  ....
  ....

- ## <u>How do you feel?</u>

  ....
  ....
  ....
  ....

- ## Record your weight: ....

Track Your Progress

Day ....   Date.................

- ## Diet Plan

  ....
  ....
  ....

- ## How do you feel?

  ....
  ....
  ....
  ....

- ## Record your weight: ....

<u>Track Your Progress</u>

Day ....   **Date**..................

- ## <u>Diet Plan</u>

....

....

- ## <u>How do you feel?</u>

....

....

....

- ## Record your weight: ....

<u>Track Your Progress</u>

Day ....   Date.................

- ## <u>Diet Plan</u>

- ## <u>How do you feel?</u>

- ## Record your weight: ....

Track Your Progress

Day .... Date..................

- ## Diet Plan

  ....
  ....
  ....

- ## How do you feel?

  ....
  ....
  ....

- ## Record your weight: ....

Track Your Progress

Day ………………… Date…………………

- ## Diet Plan

……………………………………………………………
……………………………………………………………

- ## How do you feel?

……………………………………………………………
……………………………………………………………
……………………………………………………………

- ## Record your weight: …………………

<u>Track Your Progress</u>

Day ....   Date.................

- ## <u>Diet Plan</u>

  ....
  ....
  ....

- ## <u>How do you feel?</u>

  ....
  ....
  ....
  ....

- ## Record your weight: ....

Track Your Progress

Day ....   Date..................

- ## Diet Plan

  ....
  ....
  ....

- ## How do you feel?

  ....
  ....
  ....

- ## Record your weight: ....

Track Your Progress

Day ....   Date..................

- ## Diet Plan

  ```
  ....................................................
  ....................................................
  ....................................................
  ```

- ## How do you feel?

  ```
  ....................................................
  ....................................................
  ....................................................
  ....................................................
  ```

- ## Record your weight: ....

<u>Track Your Progress</u>

Day ....   Date.................

- ## <u>Diet Plan</u>

....

....

....

- ## <u>How do you feel?</u>

....

....

....

....

- ## Record your weight: ....

Track Your Progress

Day .... Date.................

- **Diet Plan**

....
....

- **How do you feel?**

....
....
....

- **Record your weight: ....**

Track Your Progress

Day ....   Date.................

- ## Diet Plan

....

....

- ## How do you feel?

....

....

....

- ## Record your weight: ....

Track Your Progress

Day ....   Date..................

- ## Diet Plan

  ....
  ....

- ## How do you feel?

  ....
  ....
  ....

- ## Record your weight: ....

Track Your Progress

Day .... **Date**..................

- ## Diet Plan

  ....
  ....
  ....

- ## How do you feel?

  ....
  ....
  ....

- **Record your weight:** ....

Track Your Progress

Day ....   Date.................

- ## Diet Plan

....
....
....

- ## How do you feel?

....
....
....

- ## Record your weight: ....

Track Your Progress

Day .... Date..................

- ## Diet Plan

....
....
....

- ## How do you feel?

....
....
....
....

- **Record your weight: ....**

<u>Track Your Progress</u>

Day .... **Date**..................

- ## <u>Diet Plan</u>

  ....
  ....
  ....

- ## <u>How do you feel?</u>

  ....
  ....
  ....
  ....

- ## Record your weight: ....

Track Your Progress

Day ....   **Date**..................

- ## Diet Plan

....

....

- ## How do you feel?

....

....

....

- ## Record your weight: ....

<u>Track Your Progress</u>

Day ....   Date.................

- ### <u>Diet Plan</u>

....
....
....

- ### <u>How do you feel?</u>

....
....
....
....

- ### Record your weight: ....

Track Your Progress

Day .... **Date**..................

- ## Diet Plan

....
....
....

- ## How do you feel?

....
....
....

- ## Record your weight: ....

<u>Track Your Progress</u>

Day ....   **Date**.................

- ## <u>Diet Plan</u>

  ....
  ....
  ....

- ## <u>How do you feel?</u>

  ....
  ....
  ....
  ....

- ## Record your weight: ....

Track Your Progress

Day ....   Date..................

- ## Diet Plan

....

....

....

- ## How do you feel?

....

....

....

....

- ## Record your weight: ....

Track Your Progress

Day ....   Date..................

- ## Diet Plan

....
....
....

- ## How do you feel?

....
....
....
....

- **Record your weight:** ....

Track Your Progress

Day ....   **Date**..................

- ## Diet Plan

....

....

- ## How do you feel?

....

....

....

- **Record your weight:** ....

<u>Track Your Progress</u>

Day .... **Date**..................

- **<u>Diet Plan</u>**

....
....

- **<u>How do you feel?</u>**

....
....
....

- **Record your weight:** ....

LIVE

LOVE

KETO

9 781689 787871